I0094738

One Drop
At A Time

Michelle Holl

A down to earth guide to
ESSENTIAL OILS

DIY Recipes, Fun Facts
and helpful tips

SAFETY:
Essential Oils should not be used in ears or eyes, and if this occurs, never flush with water, use a pure vegetable oil instead. Some oils are classed as hot oils and may irritate the skin. Others, such as citrus oils, are photosensitive. We advise to skin test oils before use, and use sparingly as they are highly concentrated. It is advisable to keep Essential Oils away from young children and to supervise their use. If you are pregnant or have serious health issues, please seek the advice of a health professional before using Essential Oils. Always read the label.

We recommend you do your research as not all Essential Oils are of the highest quality. Feel free to contact me should you wish to find out more about the Oils I choose to use.

One Drop At A Time - Michelle Holl
First published 2020
(c) 2020 Michelle Holl

All Rights Reserved. No part of this work may be reproduced or utilised in any form or by any means, electronic or mechanical, including photcopying recording or by any information storage and retreival system, without the prior written consent of the publisher.

This book is dedicated to my three beautiful daughters, who inspire me every day to try to be a good example for our younger generations.

Essential Oils give us the opportunity to create chemical-free products that have a positive impact on our families, our lives and the Earth.

My passion is to make a difference -
One Drop At A Time.

As a mother of three beautiful girls, I have always been aware and a little concerned, that chemicals make up most of the ingredients in the products we use. I didn't really understand the extent of toxins and chemicals we use everyday.

I considered myself to live and practice a healthy lifestyle, but when one of my twins had a reaction to a beauty product, that was so serious it saw her hospitalised, I knew there had to be a better way.

DID YOU KNOW?

LABELS DON'T SHOW EVERYTHING THAT'S IN A PRODUCT .... IF THE INGREDIENT CAN BE CLASSED AS A 'TRADE SECRET' COMPANIES DO NOT HAVE TO INCLUDE ALL THE INGREDIENTS USED, ON THE LABEL!

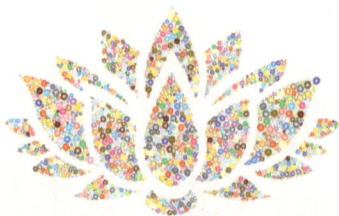

I want to educate and inspire others on how to provide a safer environment for their families.

As a hairdresser and beauty therapist for over 30 years, I was aware of the chemical dangers in mainstream products, like most of us, I used them anyway,

It was only after my daughter was hospitalised and I wanted to find an alternative to the medication they were suggesting, I did my research and discovered Essential Oils - and I've never looked back!

Later when my daughter had a reaction to Sodium Lauryl Sulphate, I realised the need to move away from the synthetically derived products on the store shelves.

That's why I created a safe alternative, making my own products at home, using natural ingredients infused with essential oils - and YOU can as well!

You'll be surprised at how easy and fun it is incorporating Essential Oils into every day life.

Together, we can make the change - one drop at a time.

With love

Michelle
xx

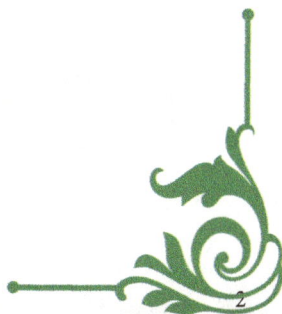

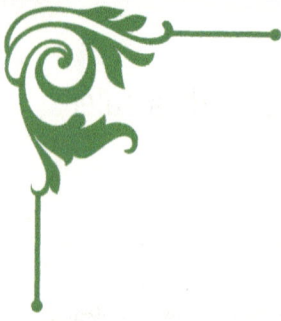

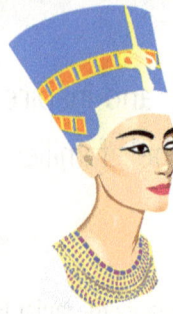

A little history...

The ancient Egyptians and Chinese have been using Essential Oils for centuries, with records dating back as far as 4500BC. Chinese empresses had an obsession for skin lighting and tightening - it seems the desire to maintain and enhance beauty is something that never fades.

The ancient cultures had many uses for Essential Oils including, medicinal, beauty, enhancing food, emotional support and embalming.

Long before commercial cosmetics were invented, women relied on naturally derived extracts and remedies. Some were so effective they are still being used today.

PLEASE NOTE:
SOME RECIPES IN THIS BOOK SUGGEST USING A THERMOMIX — IF YOU DON'T HAVE ONE, PLEASE USE A DOUBLE BOILER INSTEAD........ THAT IS A BOWL THAT SITS ON ANOTHER BOWL OF BOILING WATER TO MELT INGREDIENTS! SOMETIMES YOU MAY NEED TO WHISK TOGETHER!

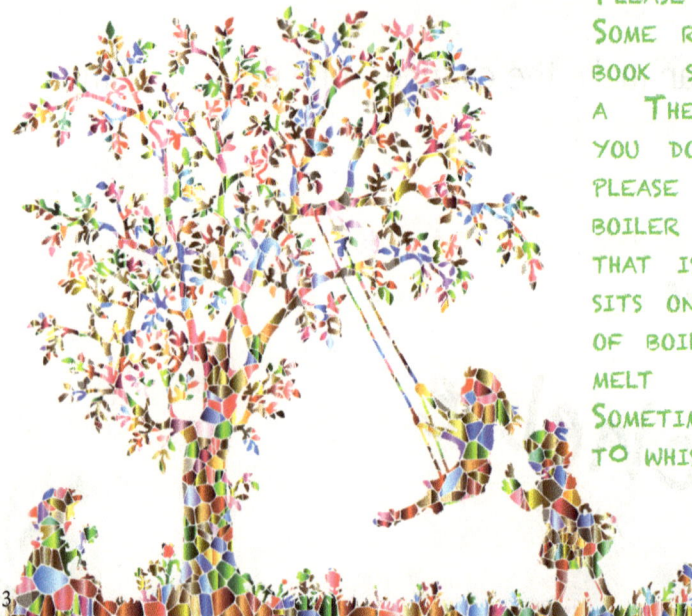

What are Essential Oils and why should we be using them everyday?

Derived from nature and carefully distilled, Essential Oils are pure extracts taken from the seeds, roots, stems and leaves of a plant - in fact all the parts of a plant. They are safe for use around our kids and pets and are environmentally friendly.

The Essential Oils are the 'life blood' of a plant, and just like human blood, they have a specific purpose to transport nutrients to nurture and feed the cells. One of the primary responsibilities of blood is to deliver oxygen to our cells. Essential Oils are documented to have the highest level of oxygenating molecules known to man.

They are made up of minerals, oxygen and amino acids and work on a cellular level. Once applied to the skin, they can enter the blood stream within 20 seconds, and affect every cell of the body within 20 minutes.

Because they work so quickly, and can impact the Amygdala, which houses our emotions, they can have a positive effect on our mood within minutes.

They are fun to work with and can be used to make an endless number of DIY products for your home and body.

In this book, you will find just a small selection of recipes and product ideas, to get you started on your own amazing journey with Essential Oils.

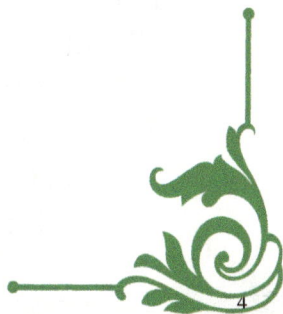

Hold Me Hairspray

Ingredients:
250ml Purified Water
1 Tbsp Sugar
2 drops Rosemary Essential Oil
3 drops Lemon** Essential Oil
3 drops Orange** Essential Oil
3 drops Grapefruit** Esential Oil
Spray Bottle

Directions:
Heat water with sugar until sugar is completely dissolved. Cool. Add essential oils. Spray.

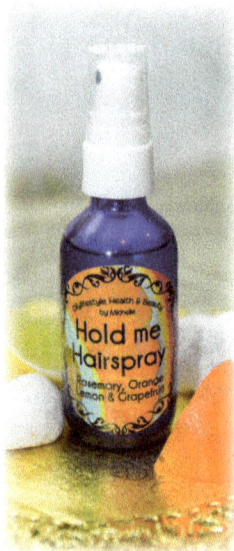

"A perfumed bath and a scented massage everyday is the way to good health"

~ Hypocrites

Super Citrus Room Spray

Ingredients:
15 drops Citrus Fresh* Essential Oil
Fill bottle with 30ml Water

Directions:
Add essential oil to a 30ml spray bottle of water. Shake before use each time.
Use as an uplifting air freshner to improve mood.

My Top 5 Essential Ingredients
– for great DIY products

COCONUT OIL   ANTI VIRAL, ANTI-MICROBIAL,
ANTIBACTERIAL.
PROTECTS AGAINST SUNBURN.
MOISTURISING, EDIBLE & TASTY.

SHEA BUTTER   ANTI-INFLAMMATORY, AIDS IN HEALING
MINOR CUTS AND ABRASIONS.
MOISTURISING.

BEESWAX   USED BY ANCIENT ROMANS AS A
SKIN SOFTENER.
CAN HELP TO HEAL MINOR WOUNDS.

BI-CARB SODA   HAS THE ABILITY TO DRAW OUT TOXINS.
ANTIBACTERIAL, ANTI-FUNGAL,
ANTISEPTIC, ANTI-INFLAMMATORY.

ARROWROOT FLOUR
NUTRIENT RICH INCLUDING COPPER
& IRON – IMPORTANT FOR OUR RED
BLOOD CELLS.
CAN HELP PREVENT ANEMIA AND
INCREASE BLOOD CIRCULATION.

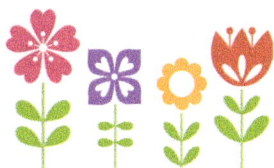

Chill Out Mummy
Body Spray

Ingredients:
2 drops Geranium Essential Oil
2 drops Lavender Essential Oil
2 drops Sandalwood Essential Oil
2 drops Ylang Ylang Essential Oil
Filtered Water
Glass Spray Bottle

Directions:
Add essential oil to bottle and fill with water.
Gently shake before use.

Did you know?

Toxic chemicals can store in body fat cells!

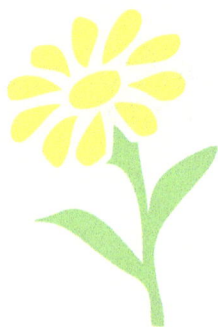

Romantic Moody
Body Spray

Ingredients:
5 drops Joy* Essential Oil
Filtered Water
Glass Spray Bottle

Directions:
Add essential oil to bottle and fill with water.
Gently shake before use.

Breathe Easy Bath Salts

INGREDIENTS:
1 Cup Epsom Salt
1/2 Cup Bi-Carb Soda
7 drops Peppermint Essential Oil
10 drops Eucalyptus Essential Oil
Top up with V6* or Coconut Oil

DIRECTIONS:
Combine ingredients but add the Peppermint oil before adding the Eucalyptus. Mix and put into jars.

Focus On Point

INGREDIENTS:
20 drops Orange** Essential Oil
20 drops Peppermint Essential Oil
Fractionated Coconut Oil
10ml glass roll-on container

DIRECTIONS:
Add essential oils and fill with coconut oil.
Apply to back of neck, on bones, directly behind the ears or roll on palms and inhale.
 Be mindful...orange is photosensitive.

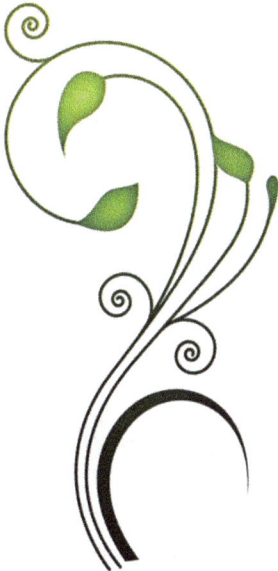

Divine Goddess

~ PERFUME

INGREDIENTS:
10 drops Joy* Essential Oil
10 drops Sensation* Essential Oil
5 drops Ylang Ylang Essential Oil
5 drops Geranium Essential Oil
V6* or Coconut Oil

APPLY TO WRISTS & BEHIND EARS.

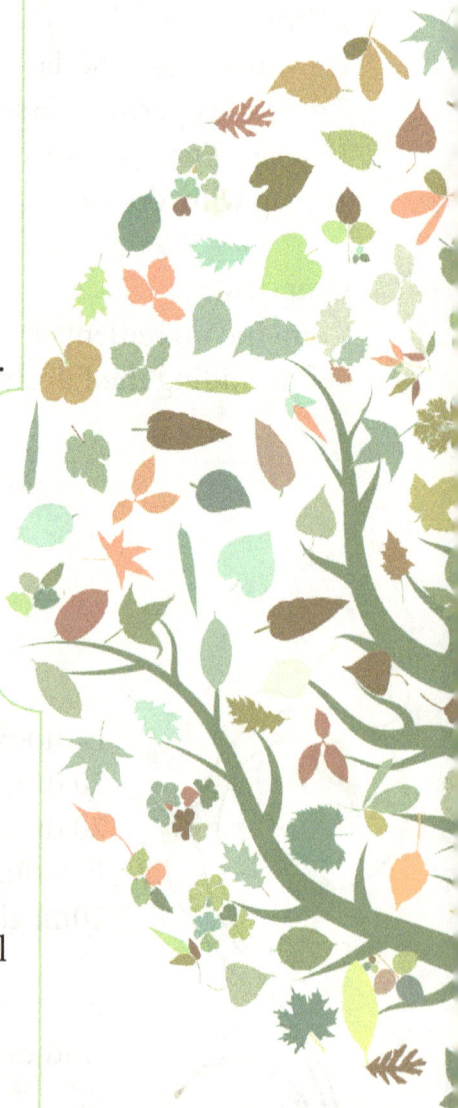

Sexy & Masculine
man'o'man

- 10ML Roller Blend

INGREDIENTS:
10 drops Cedarwood Essential Oil
10 drops Frankinsence Essential Oil
5 drops Sandalwood Essential Oil
V6* or Coconut Oil

APPLY TO WRISTS & BEHIND EARS.

'CLAP YOUR HANDS' HAND CLEANER

INGREDIENTS:
150gm Aloe Vera Gel
10ml Witch Hazel
1 Tsp V6* or Coconut Oil
20 drops Thieves Oil*

DIRECTIONS:
Mix well and put into pump or squirt bottle.

*"A day without Essential Oils is like.....
.........just kidding, I have no idea!"*

SPORTS SUPPORT

- 10ML ROLLER BLEND

INGREDIENTS:
15 drops Peppermint Essential Oil
15 drops Panaway* Essential Oil
V6* or Coconut Oil

APPLY WHERE NEEDED.

Stress Away Coffee Scrub

INGREDIENTS:
60ml ground coffee
60ml raw sugar
20ml fractionated Coconut Oil
1/2 tsp Raw Honey
10 drops Stressaway* Essential Oil

DIRECTIONS:
Mix well and put into containers or jars.

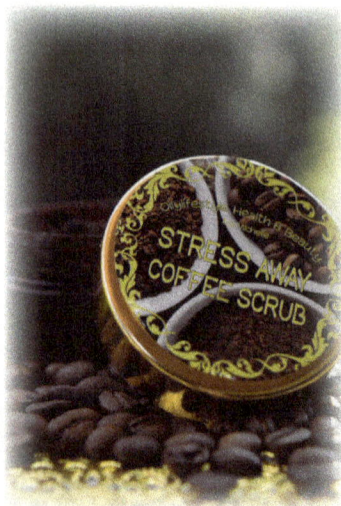

Aroma Inhaler Motivate Me

INGREDIENTS:
3 drops Black Pepper Essential Oil
4 drops Frankincense Essential Oil
3 drops Lime** Essential Oil
5 drops Orange** Essential Oil
Aroma Inhaler with wick

DIRECTIONS:
Drop essential oils on cotton wick. Place wick inside inhaler. Snap plug on bottom of inhaler. Replace cover when not in use.

"Allow things in your life that make your heart sing"
~ Andrew Pacholyk

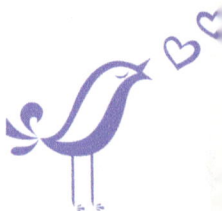

Dreamy & Jolly Body Spray

INGREDIENTS:
2 drops Bergamot Essential Oil
2 drops Clary Sage Essential Oil
7 drops Frankincense Essential Oil
2 drops Grapefruit** Essential Oil
2 drops Orange** Essential Oil
Filtered Water
50ml Glass Spray Bottle

DIRECTIONS:
Add essential oil to bottle and fill with water.
Gently shake before use.

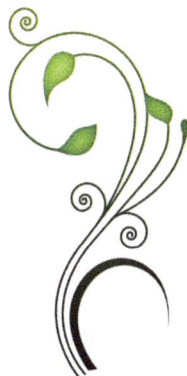

CITRUS OILS ARE PHOTOSENSITIVE

Luscious Lady Body Spray

INGREDIENTS:
5 drops Lady Sclareol* Essential Oil
Filtered Water
100ml Glass Spray Bottle

DIRECTIONS:
Add essential oil to bottle and fill with water.
Gently shake before use.

Feeling Fresh Edible Love Butter

Ingredients:
1/2 tspn Beeswax
3 tspn solid Coconut Oil
3 tspn Grapeseed Oil
1/4 tspn Agave Syrup or Maple Syrup
4-5 drops Peppermint Essential Oil
8 drops Grapefruit** Essential Oil
2 drops Orange** Essential Oil

Directions:
Melt beeswax and coconut. Add grapeseed oil and agave. Remove from heat. Add and combine remaining ingredients.

Cool It Kid!

Ingredients:
2 drops Patchouli Essential Oil
2 drops Peppermint Essential Oil
Fractionated Coconut Oil
10ml glass roll-on container

Directions:
Add essential oils and fill with coconut oil.
Apply to bottom of feet and/or up the spine as needed.

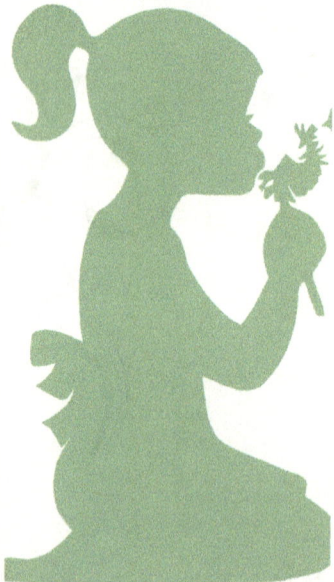

Pick Me Up

- 10ml Roller Blend

INGREDIENTS:

10 drops Eucaluptus Radiata Essential Oil
5 drops Rosemary Essential Oil
10 drops Lemon** Essential Oil
V6* or Coconut Oil

APPLY TO BOTTOM OF FEET & INSIDE WRISTS

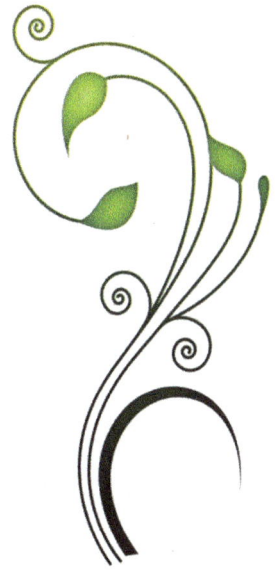

Muscle Man Mix Roll-On

INGREDIENTS:

20 drops Lemongrass Essential Oil
20 drops Copaiba* Essential Oil
20 drops Idaho Balsam Fir* Essential Oil
20 drops Wintergreen Essential Oil
20 drops Peppermint Essential Oil
Top up with V6* or Coconut Oil

DIRECTIONS:

Combine essential oils in an empty 15ml bottle and cap with a roller fitment.

Never leave home without it !

"Self care is a divine responsibility"
~ Danielle La Porte

ESSENTIAL OIL PLAY DOUGH

INGREDIENTS:
2 Cups all purpose Flour
1/2 Cup Salt
2 Tbsp Cream of Tartar
2 Tbsp Vegetable Oil
10-12 drops Lavender Essential Oil
1.5 Cups boiling water
Food Colouring - optional

DIRECTIONS:
Mix the flour, salt and cream of tartar together in a large bowl. Combine your essential oil with vegetable oil and mix into the dry incredients. Boil the water and add food colouring directly to the water. Pour 1 cup of boiling water into the mixture and stir, adding the additional cup slowly until desired consistency has been reached. Knead for 3-5 minutes until dough is smooth and perfectly squishy for play.
......hours of fun!

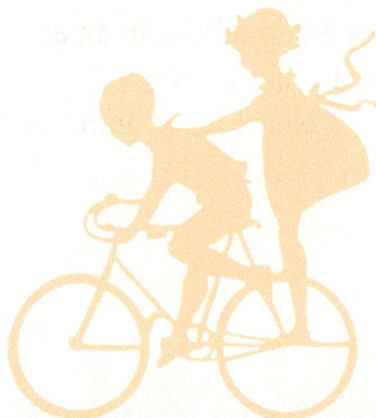

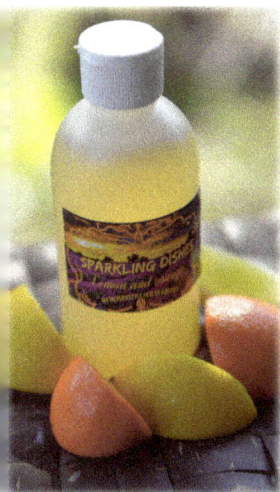

Sparkling Dishes

INGREDIENTS:
300g Castille Soap
20 drops Peppermint Essential Oil
20 drops Tea Tree Essential Oil

DIRECTIONS:
Add ingredients straight to your bottle of choice and give it a good shake, or mix in a thermomix for 15 seconds.

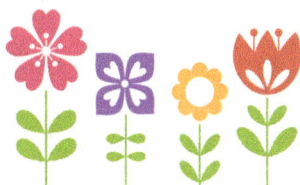

DIY Facial Toner
(ACNE REDUCER)

INGREDIENTS:
Alcohol free Witch Hazel
6 drops Lavender Essential Oil
6 drops Tea Tree Essential Oil

DIRECTIONS:
Mix together and use as an affordable astringent, with anti-inflammatory benefits.

Hip Hip Poo Ray
Toilet Spray

INGREDIENTS:
120ml Purified water
10 drops Purification* Oil
5 drops Lemon** Essential Oil
5 drops Peppermint Essential Oil
1/2 Tsp Epson Salt

DIRECTIONS:
Add salt first, then oil, followed by water.
Mix Well.

Aroma Inhaler
Keep It Clear

INGREDIENTS:
5 drops Eucalyptus Essential Oil
4 drops Lemon** Essential Oil
4 drops Peppermint Essential Oil
2 drops Rosemary Essential Oil
Aroma Inhaler with wick

DIRECTIONS:
Drop essential oils on cotton wick. Place wick
inside inhaler. Snap plug on bottom of inhaler.
Replace cover when not in use.

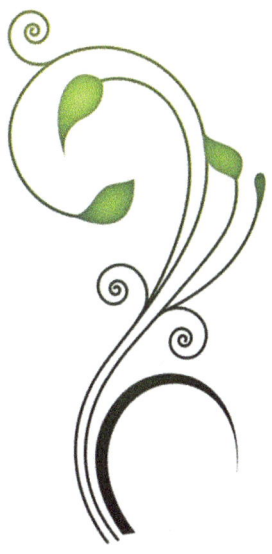

"Take care of your body - it's the only place you have to live in"

~ Jim Rohn

DID YOU KNOW?

OIL AND WATER ARE NOT BEST FRIENDS!

OIL AND WATER DON'T MIX WELL TOGETHER, SO WHENEVER YOU SEE A RECIPE THAT INCLUDES WATER, ADD A TEENY-TINY PINCH OF SALT TO THE CONTAINER OR BOTTLE BEFORE THE ESSENTIAL OIL.

IF YOU GET AN ESSENTIAL OIL IN YOUR EYES, DON'T USE WATER TO FLUSH THEM OUT — USE A CARRIER OIL INSTEAD!

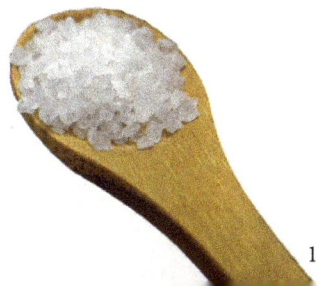

Peace & Calming

CHILDREN & TEENAGERS

- 10ml Roller Blend

INGREDIENTS:

5 drops Ylang Ylang Essential Oil
5 drops Chamomile Essential Oil
5 drops Orange** Essential Oil
10 drops Tangerine** Essential Oil
5 drops Patchouli Essential Oil
V6* or Coconut Oil

APPLY TO BOTTOM OF FEET & WRISTS

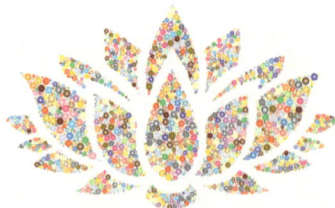

Love Your Libido

- 10ml Roller Blend

INGREDIENTS:

15 drops Ylang Ylang Essential Oil
5 drops Sage Essential Oil
10 drops Sensation* Essential Oil
V6* or Coconut Oil

APPLY TO WRISTS & BEHIND EARS.

Cool Calm & Collected

- 10ML ROLLER BLEND

INGREDIENTS:

15 drops Lavender Essential Oil
5 drops Vetiver* Essential Oil
10 drops Frankinsence Essential Oil
V6* or Coconut Oil

APPLY TO WRISTS, UNDER FEET & BEHIND EARS.

SKIN IS THE LARGEST ORGAN OF OUR BODY — APPROX. 2 SQUARE METRES! BUT IT'S VERY THIN AND WE ABSORB 60% OF WHAT WE PUT ONTO IT.

AND CHILDREN'S BODIES ABSORB 40-50% MORE THAN ADULTS BECAUSE THEIR METABOLISM WORKS FASTER, PUTTING THEM AT HIGHER RISK TO TOXINS.

ALWAYS BE AWARE OF WHAT YOU ARE PUTTING ONTO YOUR SKIN!

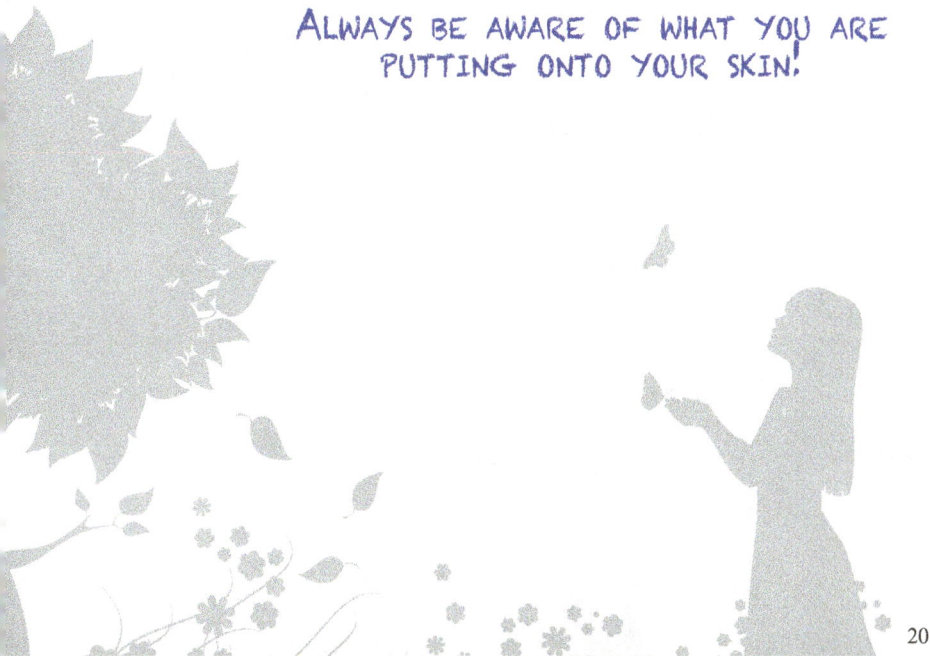

SPOTLIGHT ON....

SULPHATES

THE MOST COMMON SULPHATES FOUND IN A HUGE NUMBER OF CLEANSING PRODUCTS ARE SODIUM LAURYL SULPHATE (SLS) & SODIUM LAURETH SULPHATE (SLES).

SULPHATES ARE PRODUCED FROM SOME NATURAL PRODUCTS LIKE PALM OIL, BUT MOST COMMONLY FROM PETROLEUM AND THEY ARE WHAT MAKE CLEANSING LIQUIDS 'FOAMY'.

THEY CAN BE FOUND IN MOST PRODUCTS FOR THE BODY, AND ALSO FOR THE HOME. THESE CHEMICALS ARE COMMON INGREDIENTS IN A VARIETY OF PRODUCTS LIKE SHAMPOO, TOOTHPASTE, BODYWASH, AS WELL AS DISHWASHING AND LAUNDRY DETERGENT.

IN HIGHER QUANITITIES, THESE SAME INGREDIENTS CAN BE FOUND IN DEGREASERS AND INDUSTRIAL CLEANERS.

SLS & SLES ARE KNOWN TO BE IRRITANTS TO THE EYES, SKIN AND LUNGS. SOME PRODUCTS COME WITH A WARNING TO USE ONLY IN A VENTILATED ROOM, BUT HOW MANY OF US READ THE LABELS ON OUR EVERYDAY PRODUCTS?

THEY HAVE ALSO BEEN LINKED TO MOUTH ULCERS, HAIR LOSS, NAUSEA AND TEETH DAMAGE.

I STRONGLY RECOMMEND YOU READ PRODUCT LABELS CAREFULLY AND LOOK OUT FOR ANY WARNINGS OR RECOMMENDATIONS WHEN IT COMES TO SULPHATES!

CHEMICAL DANGERS IN EVERYDAY PRODUCTS

BODY SCRUB

HAIRSPRAY

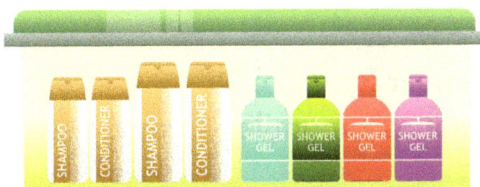
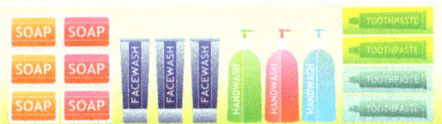
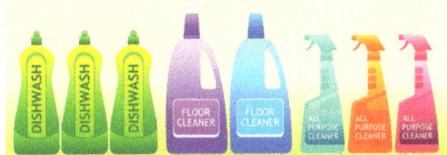
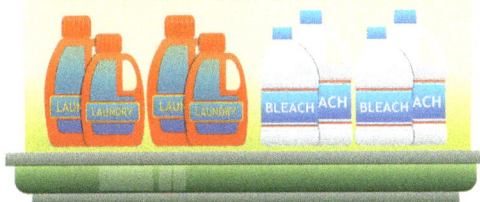

TOOTHPASTE

SHAMPOO

BODY LOTIONS

CHEST RUBS

DEODORANTS

FACE CREAM

CLEANING PRODUCTS

LIP BALM

FRAGRANCES PERFUMES

SPORTS RUBS

MOUTHWASH

Docile Doggy
Calming Spritzer

INGREDIENTS:
500ml purfied water
20 drops Lavender Essential Oil
15 drops Roman Chamomile Essential Oil
Pinch of pink salt

DIRECTIONS:
Mix all ingredients together in the bottle. Shake well before spraying.

SPRAY OVER YOUR FURRY FRIEND IF THEY NEED CALMING

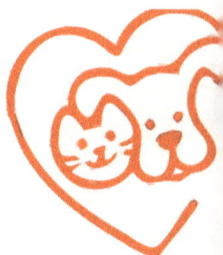

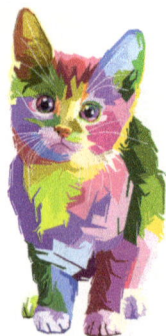

Razza Matazz
Kitty Litter Deodoriser

INGREDIENTS:
1 Cup Bi-Carb Soda
15 drops Purification* Oil
4 drops Lemon** Essential Oil

DIRECTIONS:
Shake well and place in a jar. Sprinkle over kitty litter.

Flea Be Gone

INGREDIENTS:
10 drops Lavender Essential Oil
6 drops Purification* Oil
8 drops Eucalyptus Essential Oil
300ml Purified Water
50ml Witch Hazel

DIRECTIONS:
Mix all ingredients into the spray bottle and shake well.

SPRAY OVER YOUR FURRY FRIEND!

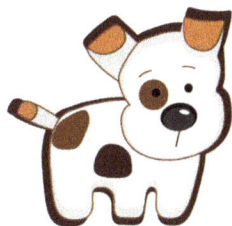

Paw Patrol
Doggy Shampoo

INGREDIENTS:
500ml water
5 drops Lavender Essential Oil
3 drops Peppermint Essential Oil
4 drops Eucalyptus Essential Oil
3 drops Rosemary Essential Oil
2 Tbsp Castile Soap

DIRECTIONS:
Mix all ingredients well in a container before pouring into a bottle. Shake well before use and lather well on your dog and rinse well.

FOLLOW WITH DOCILE DOGGY
CALMING SPRITZER

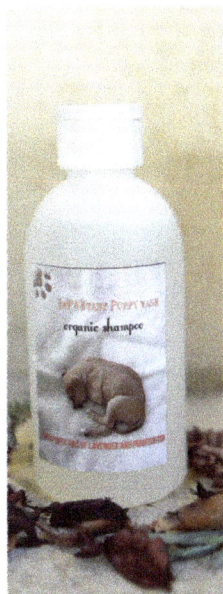

FOR OILY HAIR

INGREDIENTS:
10 drops Ylang Ylang Essential Oil
10 drops Lime** Essential Oil
10 drops Rosemary Essential Oil
60ml V6* or Coconut Oil

DIRECTIONS:
Massage into scalp 2-3 times per week. Wash out
as usual.

JOY TO THE WORLD

~ PERFUME

INGREDIENTS:
15 drops Joy* Essential Oil
10 drops Peppermint Essential Oil
5 drops White Angelica* Essential
Oil
V6* or Coconut Oil

APPLY OVER HEART OR ON WRISTS.

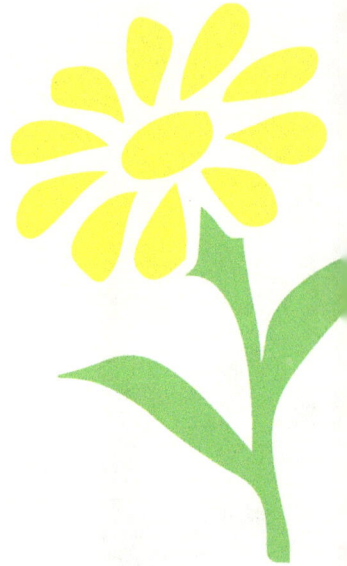

Cool & Fresh
After Sun Spray

INGREDIENTS:
70ml Aloe Vera juice
30ml Fractionated Coconut Oil
1 Tspn Vitamin E
10 drops Lavender Essential Oil
10 drops Peppermint Essential Oil

DIRECTIONS:
Mix together - place in a spray
bottle. Apply where needed.

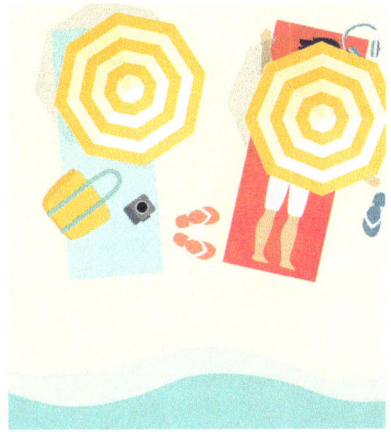

DID YOU KNOW?

IN 1928, FRENCH CHEMIST,
RENE-MAURICE GATTEFOSSE
WROTE THE BOOK
'AROMATHERAPIE'
AFTER HE HAD AN ACCIDENT AND
BURNT HIS HAND. HE PUT HIS HAND
INTO A TRAY OF CLEAR LIQUID,
THAT TURNED OUT TO BE LAVENDER
OIL AND HE WAS SURPRISED HOW
QUICKLY HE HEALED!

COMMONLY KNOWN OILS THAT ARE
NOT ESSENTIAL OILS :

COCONUT OIL
OMEGA & FISH OIL
COOKING OILS
NATURALLY OCCURRING
SKIN OILS

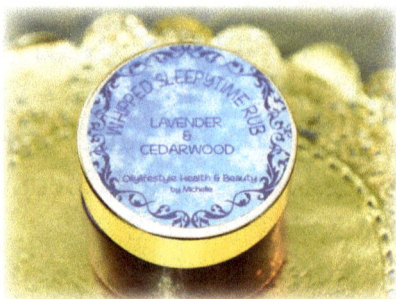

WHIPPED SLEEPY-TIME RUB

INGREDIENTS:
20g Cocoa Butter
80ml Coconut Oil
15 drops Lavender Essential Oil
15 drops Cedarwood Essential Oil

DIRECTIONS:
Add the coconut oil and the cacoa butter to thermomix for 3 mins on 90 degrees/ speed 1. Allow to sit for a few minutes. Add Essential Oils and let it sit. You want it to be firm but not too hard. Whip on high with mixer until the mixture softens and forms a cream

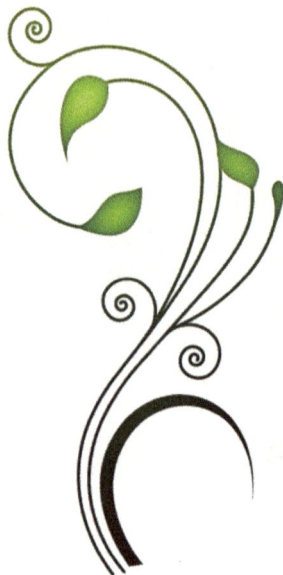

Aroma Inhaler
Rise & Shine

INGREDIENTS:
3 drops Bergarnot Essential Oil
4 drops Lime Essential Oil
4 drops Orange Essential Oil
4 drops Spearmint Essential Oil
Aroma Inhaler with wick

DIRECTIONS:
Drop essential oils on cotton wick. Place wick inside inhaler. Snap plug on bottom of inhaler. Replace cover when not in use.

Doll's 'Sigh of Relief' TempleTamer

- 10ML ROLLER BLEND

INGREDIENTS:
10 drops Peppermint Essential Oil
10 drops Frankinscence Essential Oil
10 drops Lavender Essential Oil
V6* or Coconut Oil

APPLY TO TEMPLES

"When you love yourself..... that's when you're most beautiful."

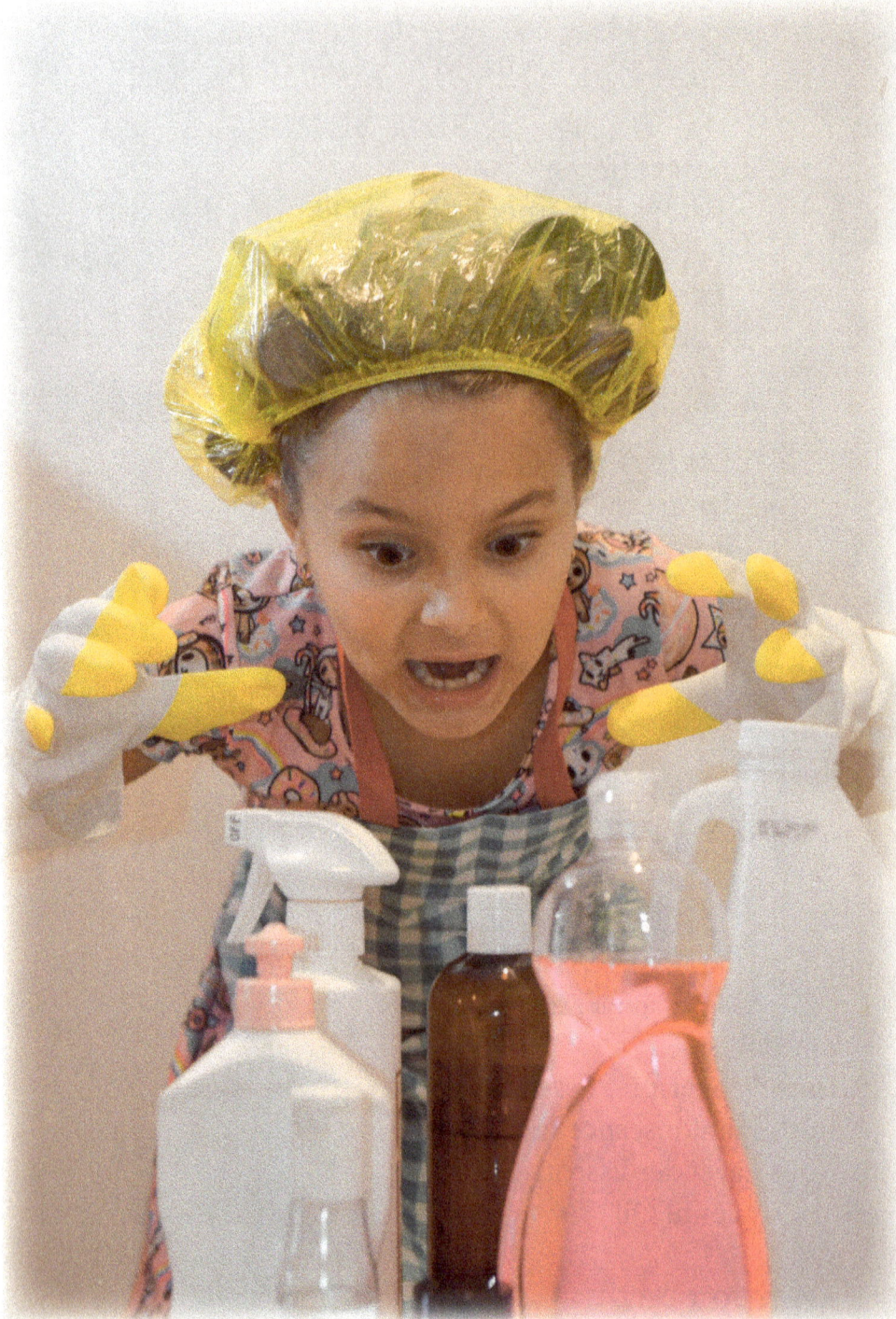

5 Crazy Chemicals To Avoid
- check labels for these toxic products

PROPYLENE GLYCOL

FOUND IN DEODORANTS, TOOTHPASTE, SHAVING GEL, SHAMPOOS, FACE CREAMS. LINKED TO RASHES, DRY SKIN AND PREMATURE AGEING.

FORMALDEHYDE — FOUND IN SHAMPOOS, BODY WASH, SUNSCHREEN & MANY MORE
- KNOWN CARCINOGEN.
LINKED TO SORE THROAT, COUGH & NOSEBLEEDS.

PARABENS — FOUND IN MOST SKINCARE PRODUCTS, GELS & CREAMS.
CAN MIMIC OESTROGEN AND DISRUPT THE BODY'S HORMONE SYSTEM.

TRICLOSAN — FOUND IN DEODORANT, TOOTHPASTE AND DISH WASHING LIQUIDS AND MORE. DISRUPTS THE THYROID AND MALE/ FEMALE HORMONES.
LINKED TO ASTHMA, ECZEMA & ALLERGIES.

FRAGRANCES — THERE ARE OVER 500 POTENTIAL CHEMICALS THAT CAN BE USED UNDER THE SINGLE NAME 'FRAGRANCE,' FOUND IN LOTS OF PRODUCTS INCLUDING PERFUMES. MANY OF THESE SYNTHETIC CHEMICALS ARE SKIN IRRITANTS, PENETRATORS AND ENDOCRINE DISRUPTORS, AS WELL AS CARCINOGENIC.

THIEVES OIL IS AN ESSENTIAL OIL BLEND BASED ON A STORY FROM AROUND THE 15TH CENTURY WHEN THE BUBONIC PLAGUE WAS RUNNING RAMPANT THROUGH EUROPE AND ASIA.

FOUR THIEVES FROM EUROPE WERE ROBBING THE INFECTIOUS DEAD BODIES OF THEIR POSSESSIONS, BUT BECAUSE THEY WERE 'USING' THIS ESSENTIAL OIL BLEND, MIRACULOUSLY NEVER CONTRACTED THE HIGHLY INFECTIOUS PLAGUE.

DIY CLEANING WIPES

INGREDIENTS:
1 Roll Kitchen Towel (Handy Ultra Double Length works well)
1 BPA-free plastic container
1 cap full Thieves* Household Cleaner
300ml Filtered Water

DIRECTIONS:
Cut kitchen roll in half and place in plastic container. Mix water and Thieves cleaner, and pour over kitchen roll. Remove cardboard from centre of roll and pull sheets from the centre. Cover with lid to retain moistness.

Pip's Crown of Glory
Hair Spritzer

INGREDIENTS:
3 drops Lavender Essential Oil
1 drop Geranium Essential Oil
2 drops Lemon** Essential Oil
3 drops Cedarwood Essential Oil
1 drop Peppermint Essential Oil
30ml Purified Water

DIRECTIONS:
Combine above ingredents and shake well. Spray onto damp or wet hair.

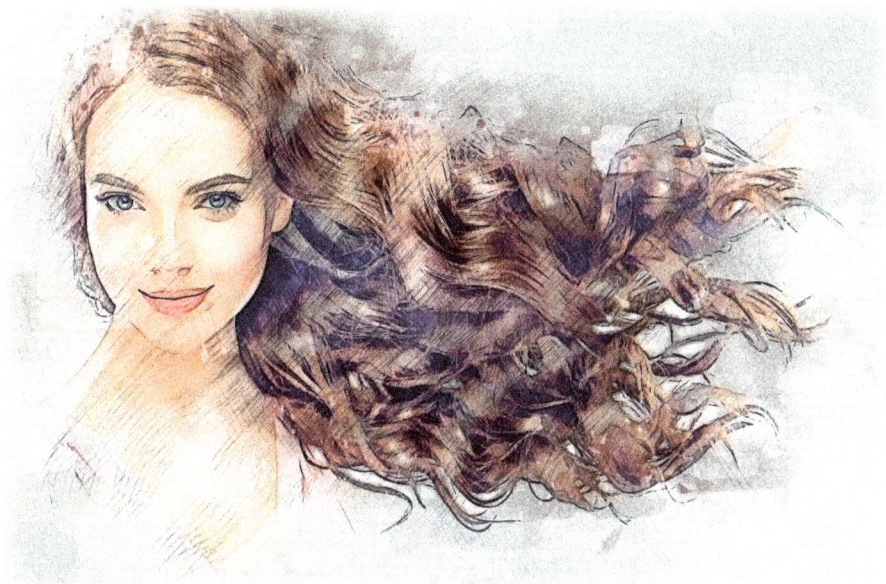

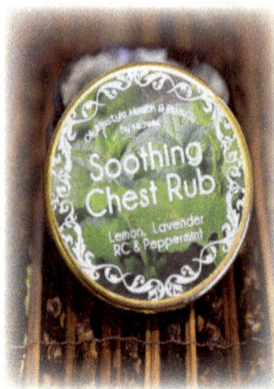

Soothing Chest Rub

Ingredients:
100g Coconut Oil
30g Shea Butter
20g Beeswax pellets
6 drops Lemon** Essential Oil
6 drops Lavender Essential Oil
6 drops Peppermint Essential Oil
6 drops RC* (respiratory comfort)
Essential Oil

Directions:
Add coconut oil, shea butter and beeswax. Melt over stove or in thermomix making sure beeswax is well melted. Add oils and mix well. Pour into jars or containers.

Household Cleaner

Ingredients:
450ml filtered water
15ml (1 1/2 cap) Thieves Cleaner Concentrate*

Directions:
In a 500ml spray bottle, combine the filtered water and Thieves cleaner.

Use to clean all household surfaces.

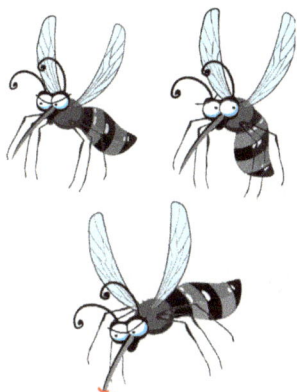

"I have an oil for that!"

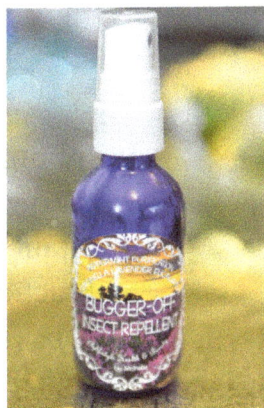

BUGGER OFF INSECT REPELLENT

INGREDIENTS:
10 drops Peppermint Essential Oil
5 drops Citronella* Essential Oil
5 drops Lavender Essential Oil
5 drops Purification* Essential Oil
20 drops Eucalyptus Essential Oil
50ml Witch Hazel
50ml Distilled water

DIRECTIONS:
Combine essential oils in an empty bottle and add other ingredients.

GUARANTEED TO KEEP THE BUGS AWAY!

Blissful Foaming
Face Wash

Ingredients:

95g water (filtered or boiled and then cooled)
45g liqued Castille soap
5g Fractionated Coconut Oil or Almond Oil
5 drops Geranium Essential Oil
4 drops Lavender Essential Oil
1 drop Frankinsense Essential Oil

Directions:

Add all ingredients to Thermomix bowl and mix for 10-15 seconds/speed 2. If no Thermomix, then mix well with a whisk.
Pour into foaming pump bottles.

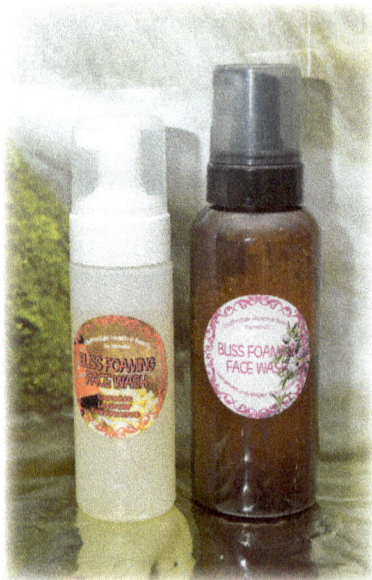

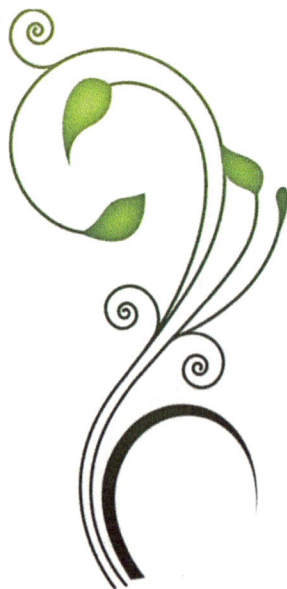

DID YOU KNOW?

THERE ARE OVER 100,000 CHEMICALS IN USE IN OUR EVERYDAY PRODUCTS — AND MANY OF THEM HAVE HAD NO 'SAFETY' TESTING!

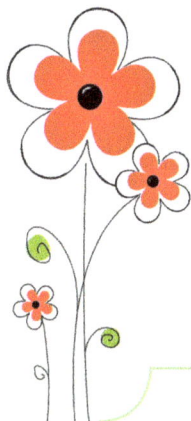

HANDY MAN SCRUB

GREAT FOR GREASY OR PAINT SPLATTERED HANDS!

INGREDIENTS:
1 cup White Sugar
1/4 cup V6* or Coconut Oil
20 drops Lemon** Essential Oil
Small Mason Jar

DIRECTIONS:
Combine all ingredients and place in Mason Jar. Add an extra tablespoon of on top to prevent it from drying out.

SCRUB DIRTY HANDS AND NAILS WITH 1-2 TABLESPOONS OF MIXTURE AND RINSE WELL.

Kick Ya Heels Up!
Peppermint &
Lavender Foot Cream

INGREDIENTS:
10g Beeswax
40g Cocoa Butter
80g Shea Butter
20g Coconut Oil
20ml V6* or Coconut oil
5 drops Lavender Essential Oil
5 drops Peppermint Essential Oil

DIRECTIONS:
Mix Beeswax, Cocoa Butter, Shea Butter and Coconut Oil in Thermomix on 80 degrees for 4 mins/speed 3 until all
melted. Add V6 Oil and essential oils. Mix for a further 10 seconds. Let
mixture come to solid. To quicken the process, place in refrigerator. Once
solid, use an electric mixer to whip for 3-4 mins or until light and fluffy.

LAVENDER IS THE MOST VERSATILE ESSENTIAL OIL AND IS OFTEN USED TO SUPPORT THE SKIN.

IT'S REFRESHING AND RELAXING SCENT HAS BALANCING PROPERTIES THAT MAY CALM THE MIND AND BODY, OR BOOST ENERGY AND STAMINA!

Put into glass jars or containers and apply to feet and heals as needed.

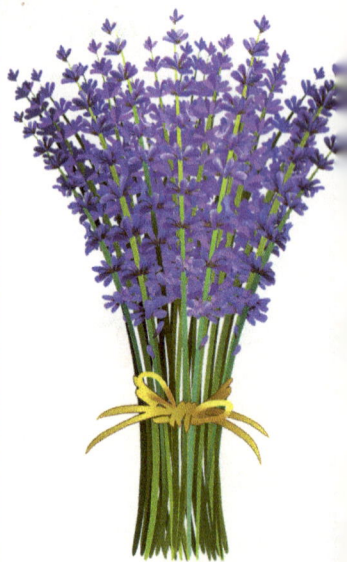

ESSENTIAL OILS ARE 50-70 TIMES MORE POWERFUL THAN HERBS! IN ANCIENT TIMES, ONLY ROYALTY SUCH AS KING TUT, KING SOLOMON AND CLEOPATRA USED ESSENTIAL OILS.

HERBS WERE GIVEN TO COMMONERS AND PEASANTS.

WHIPPED BODY LOTION

INGREDIENTS:
20g Coca Butter
50g Shea Butter
50g Coconut Oil
20g Fractionated Coconut Oil
5g Sweet Almond Oil
10 drops Tangerine** Essential Oil
10 drops Peppermint Essential Oil

DIRECTIONS:
Add Shea Butter, Coconut Oil, Fractionated Coconut oil and sweet Almond Oil to Thermomix bowl and melt 7 min/80 degrees/speed, melting all.
Add Essential Oils. Mix for 7 seconds/speed 1. Allow to cool completely - may take 30 minutes, or until the mixture starts to harden. It will go slightly opaque. It may be placed in the fridge, but do not allow to completely solidify. Must be completely cool before whipping. Whip for approx. 50 seconds/speed 4 or until creamy.
Place in containers and store in a cool dry place.

'GUMPTION BE GONE'
CLEANING PASTE

INGREDIENTS:
310g Bicarbonate of Soda
155g Castille soap
85g hydrogen peroxide (3-6%)
65g Rock Salt
15 drops Lemon** Essential Oil
25 drops Thieves* Essential Oil

DIRECTIONS:
Add all ingredients to Thermomix bowl and
mix 15 seconds/speed 5. Store in a glass jar.

Use instead of abrasive toxic cleaners.

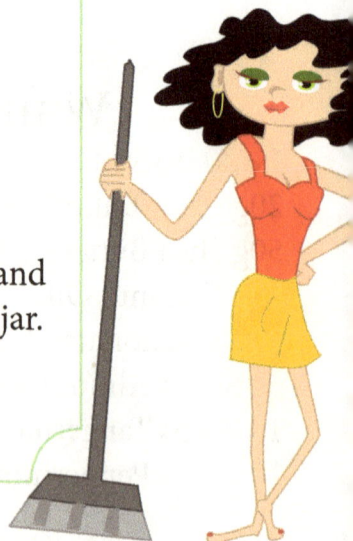

HAPPY CHEST
- 10ML ROLLER BLEND

INGREDIENTS:
15 drops RC* Essential Oil
10 drops Lemon** Essential Oil
5 drops Cobaiba* Essential Oil
V6 or Coconut Oil

APPLY TO CHEST & UNDER FEET.

FLOSSY'S FRESH BODY WASH

INGREDIENTS:
100ml Filtered Water
65g liquid Castile soap
5g Almond Oil or V6*
5 drops Peppermint Essential Oil
3 drops Citrus Fresh* Essential Oil

DIRECTIONS:
Add ingredients to Thermomix bowl
and mix for 15 secs/speed 2. Pour
    into a container.

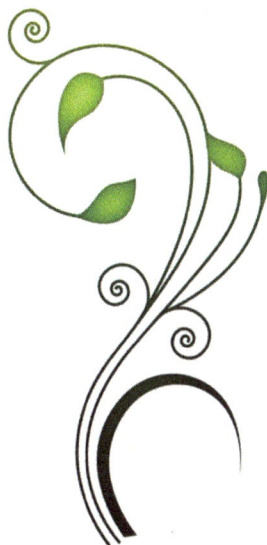

ACNE CLAY MASK

INGREDIENTS:
1 Tsp Bentonite Clay
1 Tbsp Raw Honey
1 Tbsp Sweet Almond Oil
2 drops TeeTree / or Lavender Essential Oil

DIRECTIONS:
Combine ingredients together.

Use this mask if you have oily skin, blackheads and
large pores. It deep cleans your pores and draws out
impurities.

CARRIER OILS
– Important information!

A CARRIER OIL IS A BASE OR VEGETABLE OIL USED TO DILUTE AN ESSENTIAL OIL BEFORE IT'S APPLIED TO THE SKIN. SOME OILS ARE KNOWN AS 'HOT' OILS, FOR EXAMPLE CLOVE OIL, SO ADD CARRIER OIL BEFORE APPLYING TO THE SKIN IN MASSAGE OR AROMATHERAPY!

ALWAYS READ THE SAFETY LABEL WHEN USING ESSENTIAL OILS

DILUTING ESSENTIAL OILS IS A CRITICAL SAFETY PRACTISE. BE AWARE, SOME OILS ARE PHOTOSENSITIVE AND USE IN DIRECT SUNLIGHT SHOULD BE AVOIDED FOR 24 HOURS. THIS INCLUDES ALL CITRUS OIL AND CITRUS OIL BLENDS. IT'S IMPORTANT TO TEST THE SKIN FIRST BEFORE USING.

JUST APPLY WHERE THE SUN DON'T SHINE!

MY FAVOURITE CARRIER OIL IS V6*. IT'S A BLEND OF 7 FOOD GRADE OILS, HAS NO COLOUR OR SMELL, AND IS NON-STAINING.

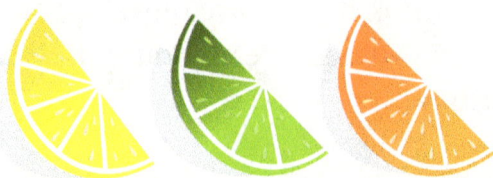

Lily's Liquid Laundry Wash

INGREDIENTS:
1/2 cup Borax
3/4 cup Washing Soda
1/2 bar of natural, organic or Velvet Soap
20-25 drops Lemon** or Thieves* Essential Oil

DIRECTIONS:
Chop up soap into small pieces or grate with grater. Melt into 1 litre of water in a pan. Put 6.5 Litres of hot tap water in a bucket and stir in Borax and Soda. Pour mixture from pan into bucket and stir. Add oil. Cover and leave overnite. Pour into bottles and shake well before use.

DID YOU KNOW?

IT TAKES 75 LEMONS TO MAKE ONE 15ML BOTTLE OF LEMON ESSENTIAL OIL.

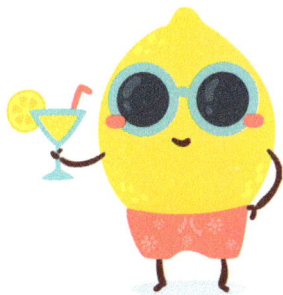

Face & Body Cream

INGREDIENTS:
25g Shea Butter
25g Coconut Oil - non fractionated
15g Emulsifying Wax
200g Purified Water
7 drops Lavender Essential Oil

DIRECTIONS:
Melt ingredients and mix well. Place in refridgerator overnight. Get out and whip into a lotion. Place in container.

Hand Cream

INGREDIENTS:
60mls Shea Butter
60mls Coconut Oil
1/4 Tbsp Honey
15 drops Lavender Essential Oil
4 drops Frankinscence Essential Oil

DIRECTIONS:
Melt the shea butter and coconut oil until they are combined. (In the Thermomix 5 mins/70 degrees/speed1). Add honey and continue to mix. Once everthing has melted and is well blended, add the oils and continue to blend.

Slightly cool the ingredients so that the mixture begins to thicken, but keep it soft. You can put the solution in the fridge for a few moments to speed up this process, but not for long. You don't want it to harden too much. Using your mixer, mix for several minutes until it has a frothy appearance, eventurally developing the consistency of lotion.

"Nothing makes a woman more beautiful than the belief that she is beautiful!"

~ Sophia Loren

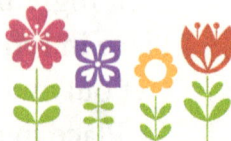

DID YOU KNOW?

IT TAKES 1 POUND OF RAW PEPPERMINT MATERIAL TO MAKE ONE 15ML BOTTLE OF PEPPERMINT OIL.

ENERGETIC & ALERT

- 10ML ROLLER BLEND

INGREDIENTS:
15 drops Peppermint Essential Oil
10 drops Clarity* Essential Oil
V6* or Coconut Oil

APPLY TO BACK OF NECK, INSIDE WRISTS, UNDER FEET.

HAPPY FEET SHOE POWDER

INGREDIENTS:
6 Tbsp Cornstarch
3 Tbsp Baking Powder
20 drops Purification* Essential Oil

DIRECTIONS:
Combine all ingredients and place into a glass jar with a lid. When needed use a tablespoon of powder for each shoe and leave in overnight. Give shoes a good shake the next morning for a fresh clean smell.

DON'T SETTLE FOR STINKY SHOES - THIS EASY REMEDY WILL LEAVE YOUR SHOES SMELLING FRESH EVERY DAY

Peppermint Lavender Bath Salts / Foot Soak

INGREDIENTS:

1 cup Epsom Salts

1/4 cup Bi-carb Soda

1/8 cup Dead Sea Salt (Optional)

15 drops Lavender Essential Oil

5 drops Peppermint Essential Oil

1 Tbsp of V6* or Coconut Oil

DIRECTIONS:

Mix all ingredients in a medium size bowl. Store in an air-tight jar and use 1/4 cup per bath.

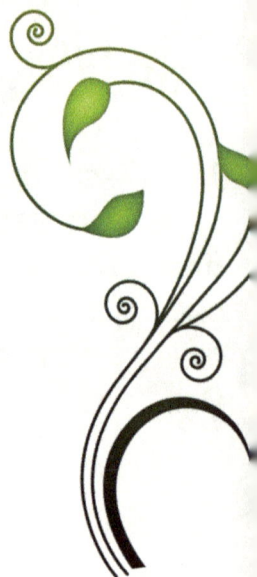

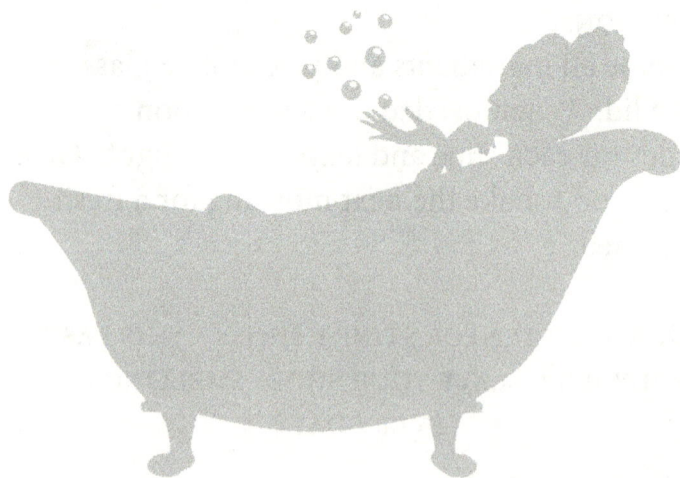

Muscle Rub

INGREDIENTS:
5 drops Wintergreen Essential Oil
5 drops Peppermint Essential Oil
80g Fractionated Coconut Oil
55g Non-Fractionated Coconut Oil
25g Shea Butter
20g Beeswax pellets

DIRECTIONS:
Add coconut oils, beeswax and shea butter into double boiler on stove top and melt all ingredients well. Can also use a Thermomix. Make sure beeswax pellets are completely melted. Add essential oils and stir well. Quickly poor into tubs or jars as mix sets fast.

RESTORE INNER PEACE AND SOOTHE TIRED MUSCLES WITH THIS BEAUTIFUL, RELAXING RUB. A BLEND OF NATURAL INGREDIENTS INFUSED WITH PURE ESSENTIAL OILS

I simply can't think of another Essential Oil I want to add to my collection.......
...... said NO-ONE ever!!

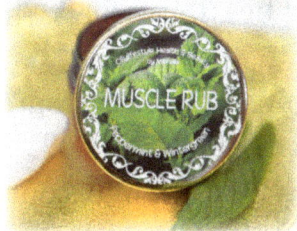

IT TAKES 27 SQUARE FEET OF LAVENDER TO MAKE ONE 15ML BOTTLE OF LAVENDER ESSENTIAL OIL.

TIGHTEN & TONE ME
FACIAL SPRITZER

INGREDIENTS:
50ml Witch Hazel
10ml Purified Water
6 drops Lavender Essential Oil
6 drops TeeTree Essential Oil
Spritzer Bottle

MIX TOGETHER!
THIS IS AN AFFORDABLE ASTRINGENT WITH WONDERFUL ANTI-INFLAMMATORY BENEFITS.

LUSCIOUS LIPS

INGREDIENTS:
20g Beeswax pellets
40g Shea Butter
70g Fractionated Coconut Oil
           or Sweet Almond Oil or V6*
15 drops Essential Oil (of choice)
        Lavender / Peppermint / Geranium

DIRECTIONS:
Add beeswax pellets, shea butter and oil to Thermomix bowl and melt. (5mins/70deg). Ensure all melted and add Essential Oil. Mix well.
Pour quickly into containers as will set fast. Can also be prepared in a double boiler.

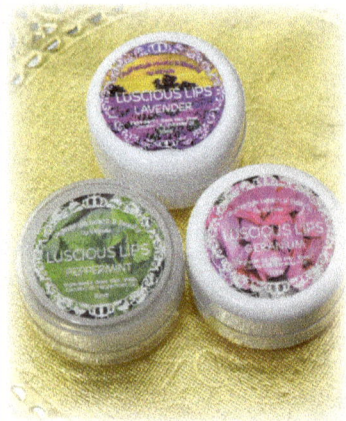

WHY USE A DIFFUSER?

DIFFUSERS ARE MULTI-FUNCTIONAL. A HUMIDIFIER, AIR PURIFIER, ATOMIZER AND AROMATHERAPY DIFFUSER - ALL IN ONE!

ESSENTIAL OIL MOLECULES SUSPEND IN THE AIR AND ALLOW US TO EXPERIENCE AROMATIC & THERAPEUTIC BENFITS!

COLD AIR DIFFUSING DOES NOT DAMAGE THE CHEMICAL STRUCTURE OF THE ESSENTIAL OIL MOLECULES.

INHALING IS THE QUICKEST WAY TO THE BRAIN VIA OUR SENSE OF SMELL.

INHALING ESSENTIAL OILS LINKS TO OUR BRAIN'S LIMBIC, WHERE WE STORE ALL OUR EMOTIONS & MEMORIES.

DIFFUSERS DISPERSE THE OIL IN A MICRO-FINE VAPOUR.

Nourishing Night
Face Balm

INGREDIENTS:

75g Fractionated Coconut Oil
55g Non-Fractionated Coconut Oil
20g Beeswax pellets
25g Shea Butter
10 drops Geranium Essential Oil
10 drops LavenderEssential Oil
10 drops Patchouli Essential Oil

DIRECTIONS:

Add coconut oils, beeswax and shea butter into a jar over boiling water, in a double boiler or Thermomix. Melt all ingredients well making sure Beeswas pellets are fully melted.When all melted, add essential oils and stir well.

WILL SET FAST SO POUR QUICKLY

GERANIUM HAS A WONDERFULLY UPLIFTING FLORAL SCENT.

ITS EXCELLENT, AROMATIC INFLUENCE HELPS RELEASE NEGATIVE MEMORIES!

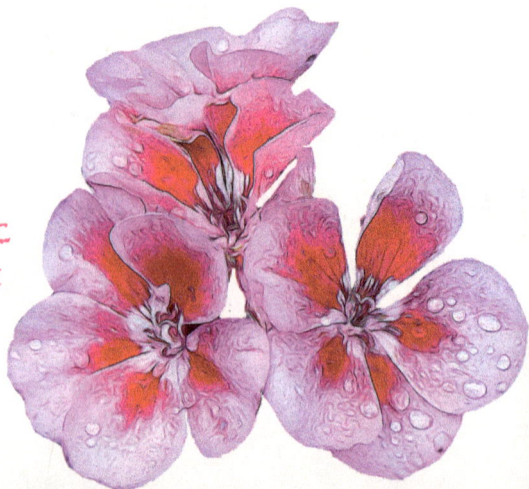

Flossy's Favourite Handwash

INGREDIENTS:
100ml Purified Water
5g Fractionated Coconut Oil or V6
50g Liquid Castile Soap
6 drops Thieves* Essential Oil
2 drops Lemon** Essential Oil

DIRECTIONS:
Add all ingredients to Thermomix and mix 20 secs. If no Thermomix then mix well with mixer. Pour into pump bottles with foaming nozzle.

USE IN PLACE OF NASTY ANTI-BACTERIAL COMMERCIAL FOAMING SOAPS

Tame The Teen Shealoe Moisturiser

INGREDIENTS:
115g Raw Shea Butter
2 tbsp Pure Aloe Vera gel
1tsp Sweet Almond Oil
8 drops Tea Tree Essential Oil

DIRECTIONS:
Add all ingredients to an electric mixer and beat until you get a fluffy mixture. Transfer to containers and keep in a cool place.

COMBINATION / OILY SKIN

There are several facts about lice that are helpful to know, as you work to get rid of them and prevent them from spreading.

Adult Lice can only live for **24-48** hours when not living on a human body.

Adult lice do not jump or fly so they can only be spread by direct contact, usually direct head-to-head contact. It is possible, though highly unlikely, to be spread by hats, hair brushes and pillow cases.

Lice Be Gone

INGREDIENTS:
10 drops Lavender Essential Oil
10 drops Tea Tree Essential Oil
10 drops Rosemary Essential Oil
60ml Purfied Water
10ml Witch Hazel

DIRECTIONS:
Mix ingredients together in a suitable container. Shake well.

SKY'S THE LIMIT
~PERFUME

INGREDIENTS:
6 drops Ylang Ylang Essential Oil
6 drops Patchouli Essential Oil
3 drops Geranium Essential Oil
3 drops Cardamon Essential Oil
3 drops Roman Chamomile Essential Oil
2 drops Idaho Blue Spruce* Essential Oil
2 drops Juniper Essential Oil
Purified Water
Vodka

DIRECTIONS:
Mix drops together in a 15ml bottle. Fill with
half vodka and half water.

ORGANIC ESSENTIAL OIL PERFUMES CERTAINLY MAKE
SCENTS!
SCENTS CARRY WITH THEM A WAVE OF MEMORIES AND ASSOCIATIONS.
HAVE FUN AND MAKE YOUR OWN!

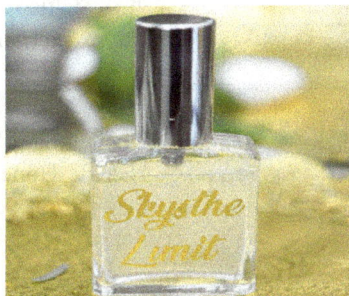

I welcome you to journey with me and learn how to make effective personal care and healthy home products that your whole family will thank you for.

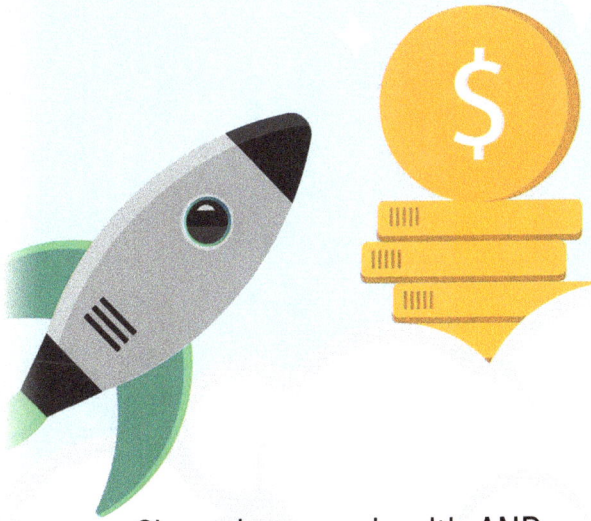

Skyrocket your health **AND** save a fortune.

If you are curious about Essential Oils, or want to know more, you can contact me at info@oilylifestyle.com.au or visit the website: www.myyl.com/oilsnbeyond

* some oils marked with one star are oil blends. Please contact me to find out more.
** some oils marked with two stars are citrus oils and are photosensitive.

Always read the label before using an Essential Oil.

Disclaimer : The information presented is for educational purposes only. It is not intended to diagnose, prescribe or treat any health condition and should not be used as a substitute for consulting with a professional health care provider.

This book has been edited and designed by Tracey Regan - All Things Writing!

If you want to write and self-publish a book of your own, Tracey can help.

You can find out more about Tracey and how she can help you at www.tregan.biz

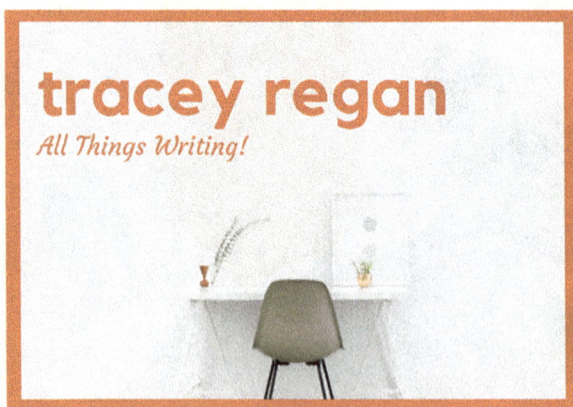

www.ingramcontent.com/pod-product-compliance
Lightning Source LLC
Chambersburg PA
CBHW062152020426
42334CB00020B/2582